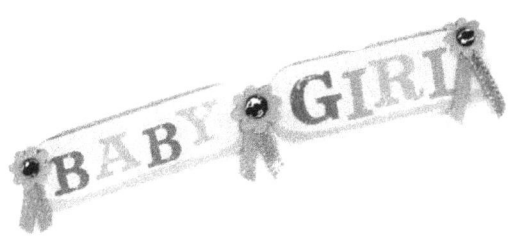

Your beautiful journey is about to begin…

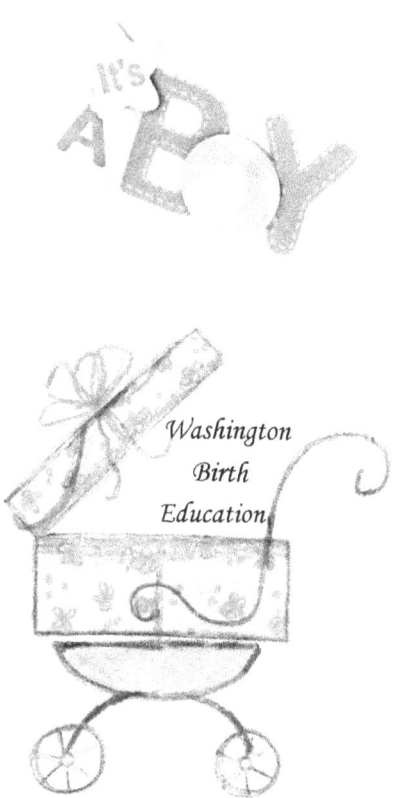

Washington Birth Education

TABLE OF CONTENTS

WELCOME TO YOUR BEAUTIFUL JOURNEY 1

CHAPTER 1: WHEN TO CALL YOUR DOCTOR 3

CHAPTER 2: WHAT TO PACK WHEN YOU GO 7

CHAPTER 3: DIFFERENT WAYS YOU CAN GO INTO LABOR 9

CHAPTER 4: VAGINAL BLEEDING 13

CHAPTER 5: PRETERM LABOR 15

CHAPTER 6: BRAXTON HICKS CONTRACTIONS 18

CHAPTER 7: WHEN IS LABOR REAL? ... 20

CHAPTER 8: I THINK MY WATER BROKE 22

CHAPTER 9: TIMING YOUR CONTRACTIONS 27

CHAPTER 10: LABOR TIMELINE 29

CHAPTER 11: BREATHING AND RELAXATION IN LABOR.............................31

CHAPTER 12: PAIN MANAGEMENT WITH MEDICATION 38

CHAPTER 13: 10 CM AND 100 PERCENT EFFACED..43
- *Episiotomy or a Natural Tear*................... 46
- *Cutting of the Umbilical Cord*.................. 47
- *Holding Your Baby* 47

CHAPTER 14: NEWBORN CARE 49
- *Is my baby getting enough to eat?*............... 49
- *More on Breast-feeding*.............................. 52
- *Bottle Feeding* 55

CHAPTER 15: A NEWBORN'S STOOL.....58

CHAPTER 16: BATHING.............................60

CHAPTER 17: SLEEPING AND SWADDLING 64

CHAPTER 18: CIRCUMCISION AND PSEUDOMENSTRUATION 67

CHAPTER 19: PROTECTING YOUR NEWBORN 69

CHAPTER 20: DISCHARGE TO HOME...71

THANK YOU..74

Welcome to Your Beautiful Journey

Becoming a parent is a blessing and a gift. During your 40-week journey, try to fully focus on the emotions and sensations of knowing there is a tiny human inside your belly—listening to your voice, developing with you the deepest, most interpersonal affection that is only known to those who carry a baby. Try to look past the aches and pains of morning sickness, fatigue, food restrictions, weight gain, forgetfulness and mood swings (just to mention a few annoying things you might experience).

Pregnancy to most women can seem to go on forever, and that includes the laboring and delivering part. Your journey, whatever path it takes you down, will be worth it. Enjoy every minute and every day with the angel or angels you bring into this world. If you have not heard this before, you will … time will fly by as you watch your baby live, laugh and grow. I pray that this small bit of information helps guide you along your way. Just remember to breathe and relax.

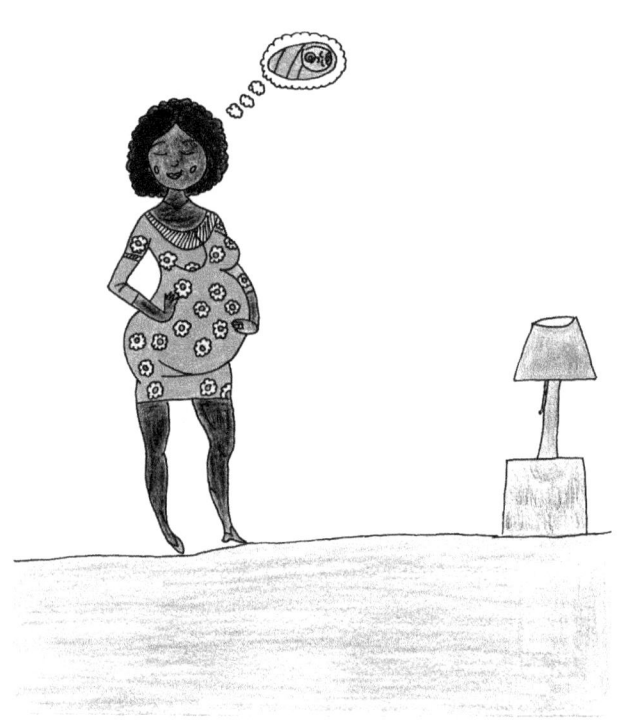

THE BIG DAY

A Practical Guide for Labor, Delivery, and more

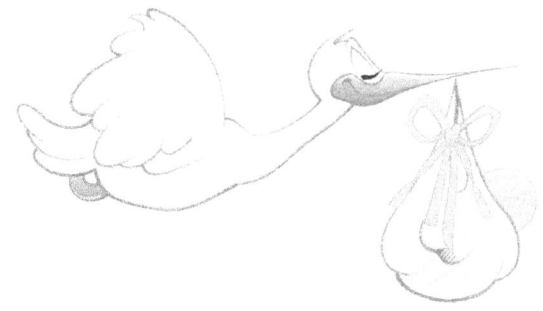

Sherri Washington
RN, MSN, RNC, CLNC
Certified Birth Instructor
Lamaze & Hypnobirthing

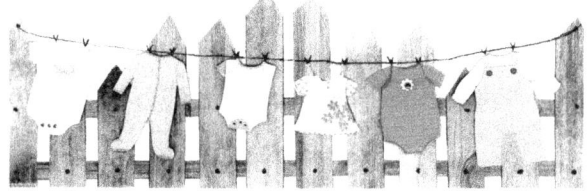

© 2019 Washington Birth Education, LLC. All rights reserved. No part of this publication may be used or reproduced in any manner without written permission from the publisher, except in the case of brief quotations embodied in critical articles and reviews.

ISBN10: 1-0959-0662-3
ISBN13: 978-1-0959-0662-0

Produced by Rebecca Barnes Media
Edited by Erin Pittman
Illustrations by Sherri Washington and Pixabay
Layout and Design by Victor Rook

CHAPTER 1:
When to Call Your Doctor

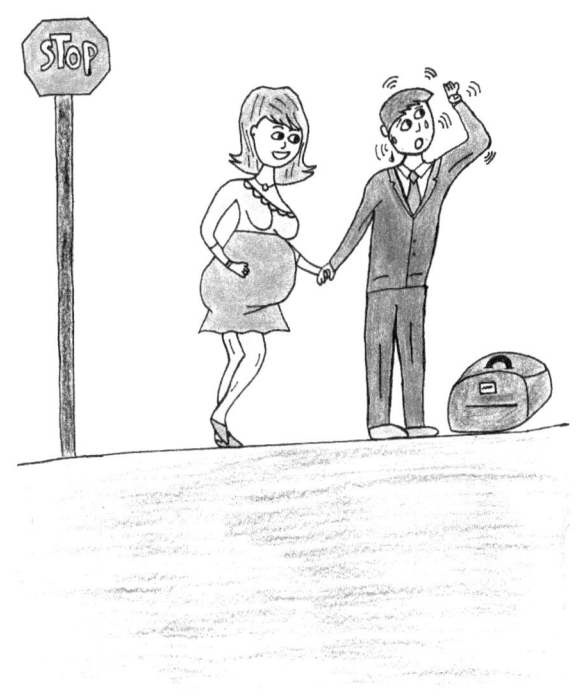

This chapter will focus on the main reasons you will need to contact your physician prenatally and when you go into labor. After you have read the entire book, you should come back to this chapter, because you will then have the knowledge to fully understand the terms and content of the things listed below, and because it is the most essential information.

*Keep in mind that these are guidelines to assist you. Your physician is available 24/7 to manage and direct your care. If at any time you have the intention of going to the hospital, always, always, call your physician before you leave your house.

Reasons to contact your doctor:

1. *You are in labor and would like to go to the hospital.* Your contractions at this point should be five to seven minutes apart, lasting 60 seconds and have continued in this pattern for at least one hour.

2. *Your "bag of water" or amniotic sac has broken.* The doctor will want to know the time it broke and the color of the fluid. Call your physician when this happens even if it's the middle of the night.

3. *You are having vaginal bleeding.* (See Chapter 4 on vaginal bleeding.)

4. *Your baby has not been moving like he or she normally does.* Your physician will guide you to the number of fetal kicks you should feel on an hourly basis. The amount will depend on how many weeks gestation your baby is. At any point, if you feel your baby is having an especially "quiet day," and you haven't felt many fetal kicks, you

THE BIG DAY

can usually increase their movement by drinking a large glass of ice water and lying on your left side for approximately 30 minutes. Even though it's tempting to reach for that Snickers bar and can of sugary soda, it's not the sugar that increases your baby's movement; it's the cold water. If 30 minutes have passed and your baby has not improved their movement, you should call your physician and share what is going on. This is not meant to frighten you, but NEVER wait on this. It is safer to be proactive rather than waiting and seeing how things go.

5. *You are experiencing preterm labor. (See Chapter 5 on preterm labor.)*

6. *You have a fever of 100.4° or higher.* If this occurs in the middle of the night, you should take 650 mg of Tylenol. Be sure to share this information with your doctor in the morning.

7. *You are experiencing burning when you urinate or your frequency has increased.*

8. *You have developed blurred vision, spots before your eyes, headaches not relieved with Tylenol, or sudden increased swelling of your hands and face.*

Remember, you have the right to call your physician ANYTIME, day or night. Please do not feel you are bothering them. Your physician wants to be aware of what you and your baby are experiencing.

CHAPTER 2:
What to Pack When You Go

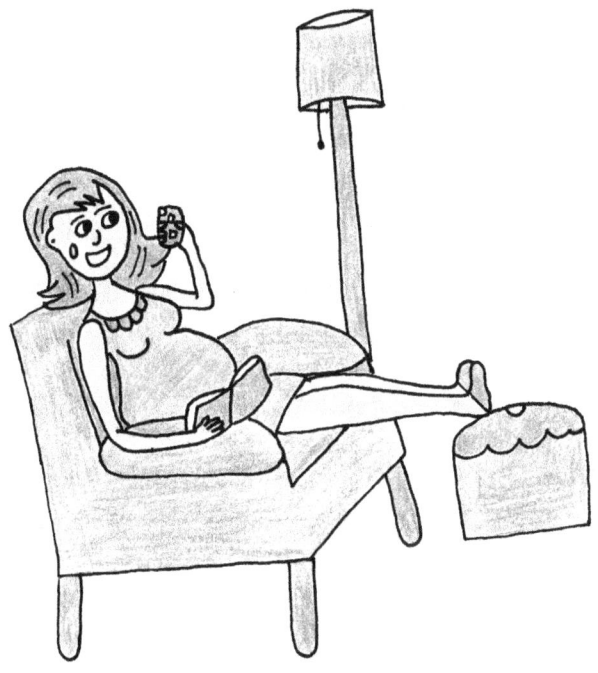

Here is a basic list of what you need to pack and bring with you to the hospital if you think this is genuinely GO-TIME!

1. **Mom needs**: driver's license, insurance card, slippers, bathrobe, pajamas, cosmetics, shampoo, toothbrush, toothpaste, device for music, earbuds, a favorite pillow, prenatal vitamins, glasses or contacts,

a picture to use as a focal point, maybe something for relaxation that smells wonderful (like lavender oil) and comfortable clothes to go home in. (You won't be quite ready for your skinnyjeans!)

2. **Your support person needs**: comfortable clothes, an extra sweatshirt and sweatpants in case your laboring wife or significant other wants the temperature in the labor room cold, toothbrush, toothpaste, more clothes (if you are spending the night), snacks and drinks, and maybe your favorite pillow. The facility where you and your support person deliver should provide sheets, blankets and a pillow.

3. **Baby needs**: an adorable outfit to go home in, a blanket for the day you leave and an infant car seat, which must already be safely and correctly installed. (Nurses are not permitted to place your newborn in the car seat or secure the car seat in your vehicle. You can call your local fire/police department, and most of them will be able to tell you days and times they are available to properly install the car seat for you.) Diapers, wipes, t-shirts, blankets and formula will be provided for your newborn while in the hospital. Be sure to have a supply of diapers and wipes ready at home.

CHAPTER 3:
Different Ways You Can Go Into Labor

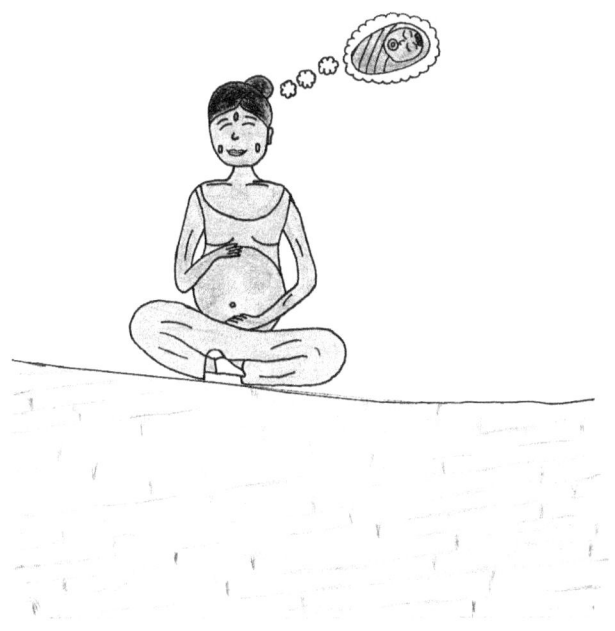

In this chapter, we will discuss the different ways that you can go into labor or deliver your baby. There are primarily fourways:

1. Around 38 to 40 weeks gestation, your brain receives a signal to begin releasing a chemical called oxytocin. Oxytocin is a chemical that when it circulates through your bloodstream will cause your uterus to contract. Oxytocin is a

naturally occurring chemical in our body. A contraction is nothing more than your uterus tightening and relaxing in a patterned manner. Most people that begin labor this way will start with contractions that are far apart and not uncomfortable. Usually, it takes hours for your contractions to become strong and regular. Later in this book, we will discuss what your physician considers to be real labor.

2. A second way you could go into labor is when your membranes rupture, or your "bag of water" breaks. The membranes can rupture spontaneously, or your physician can rupture your membranes in the hospital. Spontaneous rupture of membranes means that the bag of water will break without warning as you get closer to your due date. You may or may not be having contractions when this happens. Only 10 percent of all women will rupture their membranes spontaneously. We will discuss the other 90 percent later on in this book. We will also explain in detail, in Chapter 8, what you need to do if your membranes rupture at home or outside the hospital.

3. A third way you could go to labor is by having your physician schedule an induction. Your physician might schedule

THE BIG DAY

an induction for a variety of medical reasons. A few examples of the medical reasons your doctor might schedule an induction are: the baby measures big for their gestational age, the mother's blood pressure is creeping up too high, or you have gone up to or past your due date. These are just examples, and it is not always necessary to have a scheduled induction if you experience any of these situations. Not all women are considered candidates for induction. Induction is a way of encouraging your body to start labor and is accomplished by initiating an IV infusion of Pitocin, which is the synthetic form of oxytocin that your brain produces. This administration is done very slowly to encourage your body to take over and your body to begin producing oxytocin. Your physician will discuss this with you in detail if he or she feels you might need an induction.

4. The last way that you could have your baby is by cesarean section (C-section), either schedule or unscheduled. A C-section is where your physician will make a small surgical incision along the bikini line of your abdomen and deliver your baby from that incision. In most situations, you will remain completely awake during the procedure, and an anesthesiologist will administer medication into your back that

will make you feel numb from the waist down. A C-section is considered major surgery. If this becomes the best and safest way for you to deliver, again, your physician will discuss this with you in great detail.

CHAPTER 4:
Vaginal Bleeding

A pregnancy that is considered full term is 38 to 40 weeks gestation. If you are between 38- and 40-weeks' gestation, and you ARE contracting, you might experience something called "bloody show." The bloody show comes from cervical dilation and or cervical effacement. The amount of this type of bleeding from your vagina is usually less than a period. Bloody show, again, is typical if your cervix is dilating.

When you call your physician and talk to them about being in labor, you will need to tell them about the bloody show. If you are less than 38-weeks' gestation OR you are NOT experiencing contractions, ANY vaginal bleeding is considered abnormal, and you will need to notify your physician (day or night). Sometimes after intercourse, you can experience a small amount of bleeding; this is usually OK, but again you want to notify your physician. If you experience bleeding that is as much as a period or more than a period, this is considered heavy bleeding. If you are experiencing heavy bleeding, you need to call your physician immediately, and they may suggest you call an ambulance to get you to the hospital.

There is one other type of bleeding you may experience before you go into labor or as you are going into labor, and your physician doesn't consider this "bleeding" to be concerning. This onetime episode of bleeding (and it's not active bleeding) is when you release your mucus plug. The mucus plug is just that; it is a plug of mucus that sits inside the cervix and is blood tinged. When your mucus plug is released, you may find it in the toilet, your underwear or on tissue paper after you have wiped yourself. Losing your mucus plug does NOT mean your baby is coming, it does NOT mean labor is imminent and it does NOT mean that your bag of water is about to break. Losing your mucus plug is kind of pointless. Your physician does NOT need to know if and when you have expelled this. In fact, you might not ever even see that you have passed this.

CHAPTER 5:
Preterm Labor

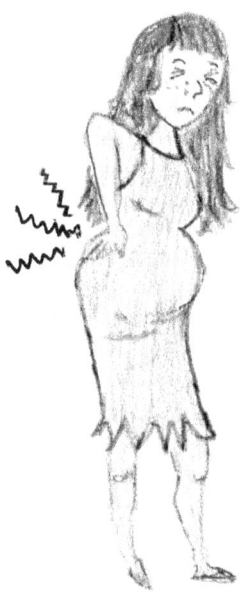

The word "preterm" refers to a gestational age of less than 38 weeks. If you are less than 38 weeks and you are experiencing any of the below symptoms, you will need to contact your physician.

Preterm labor can manifest itself in a few different ways:

1. The first way is a nagging, intermittent lower backache. This ache in your back can begin slowly and intensify over time.

The pattern can be regular or irregular and the discomfort will probably get closer together and stronger over time. Don't ignore this aching in your back; it could actually be your uterus contracting and a sign of preterm labor.

2. A second way you might experience preterm labor is by feeling cramping in your lower abdomen, just like menstrual cramps. This cramping can also be regular or irregular, and this too will probably get closer together and stronger over time. Before 38 weeks, your physician does not want you to experience rhythmic cramping or a rhythmic backache. Contact your physician if this is what you are feeling.

3. Another way you might experience preterm labor is by having flu-like symptoms such as nausea, vomiting or diarrhea. (If you are not preterm, these lovely symptoms might be signs of real labor.) But again, if you are less than 38 weeks, your physician doesn't want you to go through this.

4. Lastly, leaking of fluid from your vagina before 38 weeks is a sign of preterm labor. This leaking of fluid should not be confused with the possibility of you having an increase in vaginal mucus discharge. It is very healthy for you to have an increase in

mucus discharge. The type of fluid I'm referring to is a watery discharge that when it begins you will not be able to control the flow. The word "flow" usually is interpreted as an amount that is visibly constant, and you will not be able to stop it from coming. True, but sometimes the "leaking" of this fluid can be very slight and you might notice wetness in your underwear that is not usually there. The color of this fluid is normally clear, but it can also be green or yellowish.

5. If you think you are experiencing any signs of preterm labor, contact your physician. After talking with your physician on the phone, he or she will likely send you to the hospital. Once at the hospital, there are many things your physician can do to help slow down and even stop preterm labor.

The best way to prevent preterm labor is to hydrate, hydrate, hydrate!! If you need a number to aim for, 64 ounces of water a day is good, but more is even better.

CHAPTER 6:
Braxton Hicks Contractions

Braxton Hicks contractions are just "warmup" contractions. Your uterus is getting prepared for the big day. Some women start having Braxton-Hicks contractions as early as the second trimester, but most women will begin to have them in the third trimester. When this happens, the muscle of the uterus tightens for approximately 20 to 60 seconds and can last as long as two minutes.

Most women would not describe these contractions as painful; they can be described more like a tightening of your abdomen. So, let's differentiate when these Braxton Hicks are OK to have, and when they are not OK to have. If you are preterm, which again is less than 38 weeks, your physician doesn't want you to have more than six of these warmup contractions in one hour. If you are having six or more of these warmup contractions in an hour, then you need to hydrate with at least 16 ounces of water and rest for at least 30 minutes. If the contractions continue, then you need to notify your physician. These are probably then not just "warmup" contractions.

The situation is different if you are 38 weeks and over, since Braxton Hicks contractions can lead up to and turn into real labor. If the contractions that you're having continue to get closer together and intensify

THE BIG DAY

over a few hours, then it's very likely that you are in labor. Refer back to Chapter 1 about being in labor and calling your physician.

In review: these warmup contractions or Braxton Hicks contractions are OK to have and can happen any time from the second trimester on. If you are preterm, you should not have more than six in one hour. If this happens, notify your physician. If you are 38 weeks and over, it's OK to have more than six an hour. No matter what gestational age you are, if you are having contractions, you can try and make them go away. Drink 16 ounces of water and rest for approximately 30 minutes. Resting and hydration might make your contractions go away if this is NOT real labor. If you are in real labor, over time your contractions will continue to get closer together, the intensity will increase, and no amount of hydration or activity change will stop your contractions.

CHAPTER 7:
When Is Labor Real?

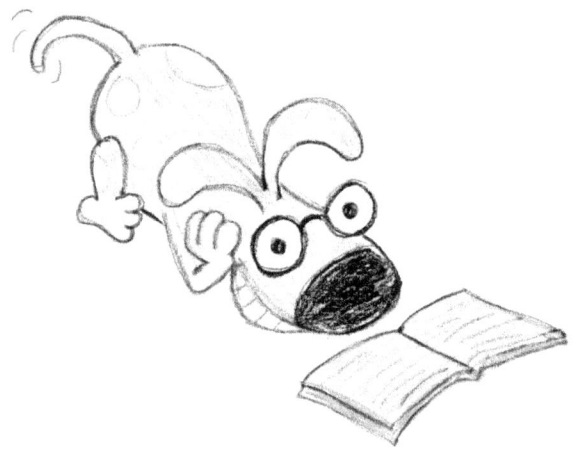

Possible labor:
Let's discuss some symptoms you might experience before true labor begins. Sometimes before you go into labor you might experience something called a "nesting urge." Basically, it is a burst of energy! You can have the urge to clean your house, clean your mom's house and clean your neighbor's house, too. Try to resist that urge to be crazy busy, because in the very near future you'll need all that energy for getting through labor.

A few other signs that may indicate that you are getting ready to go into labor are: having loose stools, feeling nauseous, vomiting or having a slight backache. Not everyone has these signs before they go into labor, and

THE BIG DAY

some women even experience a mysterious feeling that labor will begin soon. I have been told by many people who own animals that their dog or cat started acting really strange right before they went into labor.

Real labor:

True labor is uncomfortable to painful contractions in your lower belly (like a menstrual cramp) or your lower back that has continued for more than one hour. Each contraction should be lasting 60 seconds or more and should be corning every five to 10 minutes. No activity change like resting or moving around and no amount of hydration can change the pattern or the intensity of these contractions. True labor means you are having contractions that have progressed to every three to five minutes, lasting at least 60 seconds each. You can expect this to take hours. The intensity will increase to the point where you will need to use full, focused breathing to maintain your composure. One other sign of true labor is if your bag of water breaks. (Remember this can happen with or without contractions.)

CHAPTER 8:
I Think My Water Broke

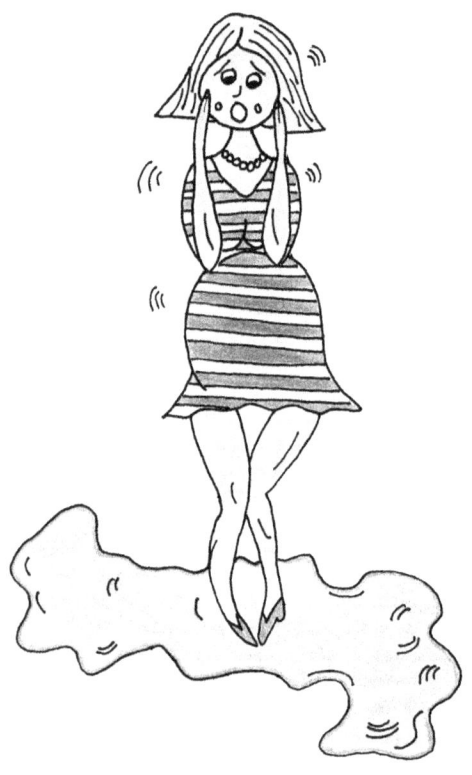

It is important to know that only about 10 percent of all women will spontaneously rupture their membranes or break their bag of water. (This means without the assistance of a physician.) The other 90 percent will have their membranes ruptured by a physician in the hospital. Rupturing your membranes can

THE BIG DAY

happen with or without contractions.

It does not hurt to have your membranes ruptured by your physician, as the membranes themselves have no nerve endings. Your physician will complete this procedure in the hospital, by using a small thin instrument called an amniotic hook. Once your membranes have ruptured, you will continue to leak amniotic fluid until the delivery of your baby. There can be a lot of fluid in there; at term, a fetus can be surrounded by approximately 600 ml of amniotic fluid.

There are a few reasons why your physician may choose to rupture your membranes. The first reason is that sometimes during labor when you are contracting, the bag of water acts as a cushion between the baby's head and your cervix. This cushioning lessens the force of the baby's head against the cervix and dilation of the cervix is slower to progress. A second reason the physician might want to break your bag of water is it's important that the physician knows the color of your amniotic fluid.

Let's discuss the different colors the amniotic fluid might be. As health care providers, our favorite color is clear or pinkish clear. Your baby enjoys floating around in, drinking and breathing the clear amniotic fluid. Yes, in-utero your baby is actually a water breather. (They get their oxygen from the umbilical cord, not their lungs like we do.) There are times, and it happens quite frequently, when your baby might have a bowel movement inside the amniotic sac, which changes the fluid from clear to green, yellow or brown. (Yuck!) But no worries, as long as you follow the "When to Call Your Doctor Rules," (# 2) it will be OK. Your physician doesn't really know why some babies have their first bowel movement inside the womb instead of waiting until the outside, but it is nothing you have done as the mom that causes this to happen. Knowing what color the fluid is can be important, since it helps us prepare for your delivery.

But what if you are among the group of women who spontaneously rupture their membranes? Then you are part of the 10 percent club! Let's discuss the sequence of events that will occur if you do rupture your membranes outside the hospital.

Remember, this can happen with or without you experiencing contractions. When your water breaks, it will either come with a large gush or a slow trickle. Again, both can be without warning. When a large gush occurs, there is nothing you can do to stop the fluid or slow it down. Crossing your legs tightly, doing a Kegel squeeze or standing on your head will not prevent the water from continuing to leak.

The water will continue coming out until your baby is born, so have some large pads on hand at home and put one on. Note the time your water broke, the color of the fluid and

THE BIG DAY

then call your physician. Your physician will want to know when this has occurred even if it's in the middle of the night. After talking to your physician on the phone, he/she will probably have you head to the hospital. Please remember to ALWAYS call your physician first before going to the hospital.

Sometimes it can be a little tricky to determine if your membranes have ruptured, because it might not come out in a large gush. Sometimes it comes out in the little trickle. If your water starts leaking and is a little trickle, your physician will want you to do a few things before calling.

1. Go to the bathroom and empty your bladder.
2. Pat yourself dry with toilet paper.
3. Place a clean, dry pad in your underwear.
4. Walk around for 30 minutes or so. If your pad becomes even a little wet, then your water probably has broken, and you will need to call your physician. If the pad is not wet, then it is very likely that your membranes have not ruptured.

Remember that your bladder sits down low where the baby can sometimes punch or kick it, and then, unfortunately, you might release a little urine. Sometimes your urine is clear because you've been consuming a lot of water. When this happens, it might be hard for you to tell if the leaking is urine or amniotic fluid. No worries, though. After you call your physician and he/she has met you at the hospital, there is a simple test that can be done to help determine if you really did break your bag of water or if your baby just punched your bladder.

Points to remember:

1. Note the time and color of the fluid if you think your bag of water has broken.

2. Call your physician as soon as you notice fluid leaking. (Remember that you might need to do the "bathroom pad trick" before you call.)

Clear, pink-tinged,
light green, dark green,
light yellow, dark yellow,
blood-tinged, rainbow. (just kidding)

No worries. Just call your physician.

CHAPTER 9:
Timing Your Contractions

There are two important aspects when it comes to timing your contractions.

1. DURATION - Duration is defined as how long a single contraction lasts from when it begins to when it ends. The timing on this should occur in intervals of seconds, usually 60 to 90.

2. FREQUENCY - Frequency is defined as how often contractions are happening. We time frequency from the beginning of one contraction through the rest period, to the beginning of the next contraction. This timing should occur in minute intervals; this can vary depending on where you are in your labor progression. Frequency can be anywhere from every 15 minutes to "really" being in labor, contracting every three minutes.

In the very beginning of your labor, it is not necessary to keep track of every contraction you have. The reasons for this are you will drive yourself crazy and your contractions might subside and go away.

So, at what point is it OK to start keeping track of the duration and frequency of your contractions? Well, everyone is different, and your physician does not want to know, nor does he or she want you to keep a tally of every single contraction. Most women start keeping track of and timing their contractions when the contractions are occurring every seven minutes or so, are lasting 60 seconds in duration and have been in this pattern for at least one hour. At this point, your contractions probably will be moderately uncomfortable.

You should start keeping track of your contractions when they become moderately uncomfortable. When your contractions are five to seven minutes apart, lasting 60 seconds and occurring in this pattern for at least one hour, it's time to call your physician.

I need to share with you that you can also get an app on your phone that will time your contractions, and, with just a push of a button, it will give you a summary of the duration and frequency of your contractions.

CHAPTER 10:
Labor Timeline

A. You started contracting and are waiting for your contractions to become regular. This time varies widely and can take from two to six hours.

B. You have now progressed to having regular contractions. You are contracting every five to seven minutes, and your cervix is dilating. You are now in labor. This is the first stage of labor, called the Early Phase. The Early Phase is unpredictable and can vary from a few hours to many hours. Your cervix will dilate from 1 cm to 3 cm.

C. Once you are 3 cm dilated, you are still in the first stage of labor, but are now considered to be in the Active Phase of labor. Your cervix will dilate from 3 cm to 7 cm. At this point you should continue to dilate 1 cm every hour. The Active Phase can last 4 to eight hours.

D. Still in the first stage of labor, but now in the Transition Phase. Your cervix will dilate from 7 cm to 10 cm. This last phase can take 3 to five hours.

E. The second stage of labor now begins. Your cervix is 10 cm dilated and 100 percent effaced. The second stage is the "pushing stage." You will actively push your baby down the birth canal with every contraction you have. Here is where you must have saved your strength and energy; here's where the hard work comes in. This stage may take from 30 minutes to two hours. This stage ends when your baby is out!

F. The third stage of labor is the release of your placenta. Approximately three to five minutes after your baby is delivered, you will push one more time, and your placenta will be delivered. It is not hard to push the placenta out; it takes very little effort.

G. The fourth and final stage of labor is the Recovery Stage. At the beginning of this stage, you and your baby will be monitored closely for about two hours. During these two hours, your nurses are going to assist you with breast-feeding, if you choose to do so. You will be given something to eat and will be offered pain medicine if needed. Enjoy this very special time!

Duration of each stage:

A	B	C	D
2 -6 hrs.	Uncertain	4-8 hrs.	3-5 hrs.
E	F	G	
30 min.	3- 5 min.	2 hrs.	

CHAPTER 11:
Breathing and Relaxation in Labor

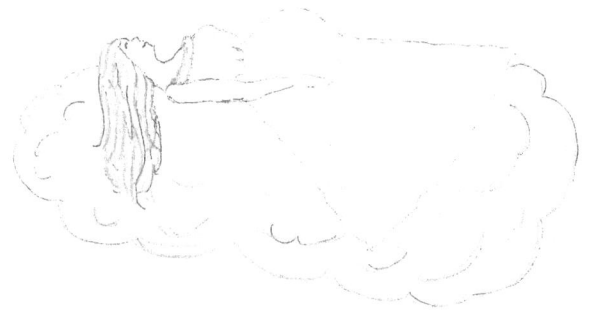

In this chapter, I'd like to share some techniques for breathing and relaxation that, in my 25 years of being a labor and delivery nurse, I have used to assist patients. I have a certification in Inpatient Obstetric Nursing, Lamaze and Hypnobirthing. I will use all these together as the fundamental concepts that will be a part of this chapter.

Whatever ends up being your method of child birth, and there are many, BREATHING and RELAXATION are key. When your contractions have progressed to the point where you are no longer smiling, it is important that you begin using a relaxed, focused breathing technique. Relaxed focus breathing is merely breathing in through your nose, full, deep and slowly, then blowing out through your mouth, full, deep and slowly. You and your support person should count from one to 10 during the entire duration of each contraction.

At the beginning of each contraction, start with a full breath in (through your nose) and a full breath out (through your mouth) at a moderate pace. This is called a cleansing breath, and you want to start each contraction cycle with a cleansing breath. After one cleansing breath, you move into relaxed focus breathing.

So, relaxed focus breathing goes like this:

You feel your contraction beginning to start, and you take a cleansing breath, in and out. As if to say in your mind, "OK, let's get this party started." Your support person will then say "one," and you will begin your focused breathing. Take a full, deep breath slowly in through your nose, and exhale that full deep breath slowly out through your mouth. Then your support person will say "two," and you will take a full, deep breath slowly in through your nose, and exhale that full, deep breath slowly out through your mouth. Your support person will then say "three," and you will take a full, deep breath slowly in through your nose, and exhale that full, deep breath slowly out through your mouth. This cycle of counting and breathing will continue until that one contraction is

THE BIG DAY

over. (Usually, your support person has counted from one to 10, and you have completed breathing in and out 10 times. Anywhere from 60 to 90 seconds will have gone by.)

You completely relax and breathe normally in between your contractions. This counting and focused breathing is amazing in getting you through one contraction at a time.

Breathing is a distraction for you, but for your baby, your relaxed focus breathing is essential! When you are experiencing contractions and your belly or uterus becomes hard, the blood flow to your baby is diminished. During your contraction, if you are breathing well, then we can assume that YOUR blood is being well oxygenated. When your contraction is over and your baby is no longer being squeezed, then the blood that flows from your vessels through the placenta and umbilical cord to your baby will also be well oxygenated, resulting in a happy, happy baby.

Review the following chart for relaxed focused breathing:

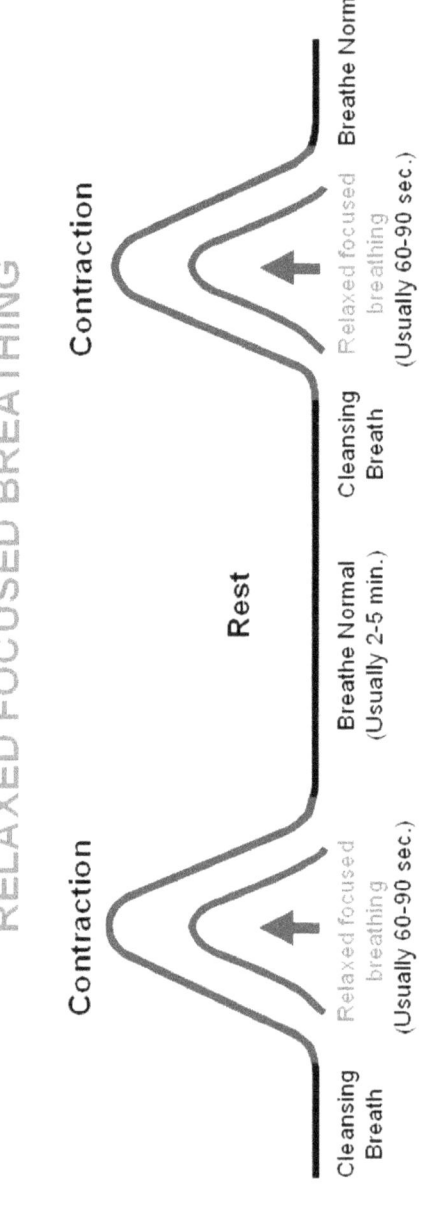

THE BIG DAY

Music: melody or harmony; any succession of sounds so modulated as to please the ear. Most facilities will allow any electronics in your birthing room. Just have this prepared ahead of time on your laptop, iPhone, CD player, etc. Whatever your choice of music is, you need to compile a few hours' worth (at least 8hrs) of your favorite tunes. Music is another distraction that will help occupy your mind as you are progressing through labor. You can play your music in labor and delivery by using any means as mentioned above. I do recommend having a pair of earbuds to add yet another distraction for you while in labor.

In review, the average contraction lasts approximately 60 seconds. If your support person is counting for you from one to 10 repeatedly as you are using your focused breathing technique, then every time you hear the number 10 being whispered, you can reassure yourself that the contraction is nearly over or IS over.

Your support person will also need to monitor the speed of your breathing. When we become uncomfortable, we tend to hyperventilate, (breath too fast) or hypo ventilate (breath too slow). The support person plays a vital role in watching the person in labor. Support persons must selectively keep an eye on your breathing, ensuring it is calm, full and regular; your hands, which need to be relaxed and still; your face, which should show an expression of peacefulness; and your shoulders, which should remain down and relaxed. It would be helpful before you go into labor for you to show your support person an example of your, "I'm stressed and in pain" facial expression and your "I'm relaxed and floating on a cloud" facial expression. My husband said that sometimes he couldn't tell the difference.

When your contractions are strong enough to dilate your cervix, and labor is progressing, you will need to put all these tools (relaxation and breathing techniques) together. By this point, you might be sitting in a rocking chair in your labor room or walking in the halls. You have one earbud in so you can hear your beautiful music, and the other ear is attentively listening to your support person coaching you through the counting of 1 to ten. You are breathing slowly, and you are relaxing every muscle in your body. Your shoulders, hands, face and all the way down your body are relaxed. You are concentrating on listening.

Now add one more thing. I want you to visualize something beautiful. You can have your eyes open looking at something like a picture or someone, or you can close your eyes and imagine the waves and tide of a turquoise-colored tropical ocean. I love the ocean idea, so I pictured myself standing on a warm, pure-white sandy shore, gazing out as the tide came in and out, in

THE BIG DAY

and out just as you are breathing in and out.

Another visualization technique you might like is to picture yourself floating on a cloud, lying on your back with your arms stretched out wide, feeling nothing but the cushion of air. Your mind will be so occupied by the music, the counting, the breathing, the relaxation and the visualization that you won't have time to think about anything else. Just breathing and staying RELAXED.

Your support person will need to remain relaxed too. Your support person's voice should be soft, slow and soothing. It is the job of the support person to remind you to keep all your muscles limp and lose. It also might be possible while you're in labor to get into a Jacuzzi tub or sit on a bench in the shower. This will be up to your physician. However, if you can use warm water in any form, this can take your relaxed body to a new level and will facilitate total relaxation of your body and the dilation of your cervix.

CHAPTER 12:
Pain Management with Medication

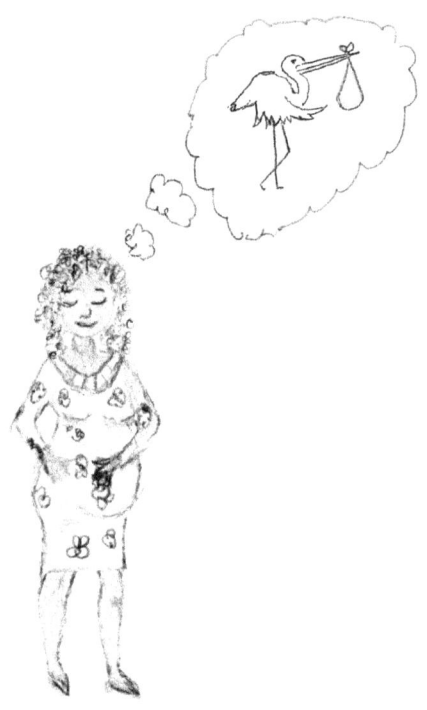

It is very important for you to keep an OPEN MIND about the labor and delivery experience that you wish to have, and the labor and delivery experience you will have. We need to be honest about the fact that not all women are able to go through labor and deliver their baby without pain

THE BIG DAY

medication. In fact, there are circumstances beyond your control when accepting pain medication could facilitate your delivery.

For example, if the duration of your labor has gone on longer than you expected and you have exhausted every bit of your strength, IT'S OK to use pain medication during labor and delivery. I know with all my heart that the end goal that you and your support person have is the EXACT same goal that your obstetrician has—the HEALTH AND SAFETY OF YOUR BABY AND YOU!

There are a few types of medications that can be administered through your IV that have a temporary effect but can be very helpful if you just need an hour or so of pain relief. Your physician can discuss these medications with you and make you aware of the most beneficial time to obtain them. Any medication you receive through your IV will, in different amounts, go to your baby. Most of these medications will begin to diminish your pain immediately.

You will be told that right after receiving one of these medications you will need to stay in bed for the duration that the medication lasts, about an hour or so. These medications will make you feel drowsy, and the baby will likely nap while you're napping. We know this because your baby's heart rate will demonstrate a tracing that is indicative of a sleeping baby. Again, your physician would not order these types of medications if it were not safe.

An example of an IV pain medication is Stadol. There are other IV pain medications that can be given at the discretion of your doctor. Another type of pain medication that might be available to you is laughing gas or nitrous oxide. Nitrous oxide is usually self-administered and is not available in all facilities. Please understand that any of the above-mentioned medications are up to the discretion of your obstetrician, and it is possible that they might have something completely different to offer you. Another type of pain management is an epidural.

Epidurals are used widely for many different procedures where pain management is required. When we use epidurals during labor and delivery, as with the above-mentioned forms of pain management, it is considered safe for mom and baby.

Epidurals are used and appreciated because they can give pain relief to laboring women without affecting their cognition, and they are not administered via mom's blood stream; therefore, the medication does not go directly to the fetus. The results are a mentally alert, laboring mom, free from contractions that are painful. Happy face!

At the point in your labor when your cervix is dilating, you should be able to ask your physician for an epidural. Some physicians like their patients to be dilated a certain

THE BIG DAY

amount before offering an epidural. I can't give you an exact time on when you should or could get your epidural, because every physician is different and it will be at their discretion. I can tell you that there is a huge window of opportunity to get the epidural.

An anesthesiologist is the doctor who places epidurals. When you are in labor you will have an opportunity to speak with the anesthesiologist. At that point, he/she will go over the process of getting an epidural, the risks, the side effects and the benefits. I can briefly explain the procedure from two perspectives, the perspective of a labor and delivery nurse and the perspective of a patient, from being one myself and having received two epidurals.

You will be asked to either sit up on your bed with your legs dangling over the side or lie on your side in a fetal position. Your lower back is numbed with a small needle and some numbing medication. A second needle is then placed into your back where you were just numbed, and a really thin catheter is threaded into a space in your back called the epidural space. Needles are not left in your back, just a very small catheter where a liquid medication can be continuously infused. The medication will only wear off if the infusion is stopped. Getting an epidural usually takes about 10 minutes and then it takes another 15 to 20 minutes for you to feel the full effects of the medication. Once it is in place, most facilities will require you to do two things.

First, because your legs will be weak, you will be asked to stay in bed. And secondly you might be told that a Foley urinary catheter will need to be placed into your bladder to keep it empty and facilitate the decent of your baby's head into the birth canal. I want to share with you that there are some birthing centers and hospitals that allow you to walk around after you get your epidural, but that is very dependent upon where you are actually delivering. Your epidural will stay in place, because it will be secured to your back with lots of tape — I mean lots of tape! You will receive a complimentary back waxing when the tape is removed! In most facilities, the epidural is turned off right after you deliver your baby. It normally takes about two hours for the medication to wear off and for your legs to be strong enough for you to be able to walk to the bathroom with assistance. After approximately two hours, your nurse will remove the tape from your back, and the epidural catheter will slide out. You will not feel the catheter being pulled out, BUT you might feel the tape coming off your back.

CHAPTER 13:
10 cm and 100 Percent Effaced

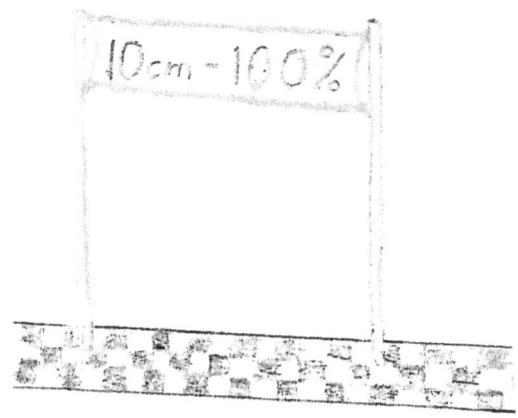

If you have chosen not to have an epidural for your labor and delivery experience, there might come a time when you would need to utilize one last breathing technique. This technique is used when you are close to 10 cm dilated but not quite ready to push. Without an epidural, as you approach 10 cm, your body will automatically have the urge to bear down in your rectum and push. It feels exactly like having to move your bowels. This urge to push is uncontrollable, and slow breathing becomes impossible.

At this point, your labor nurse or your physician will be right there with you. The idea behind this different breathing technique is to encourage you to breathe out in short, quick breaths during your contraction instead of slow, focused ones. During your contraction, you will say the words, "Hee, hee, hee, hee," then blow out the remainder of the air, like blowing out a candle. Then quickly again say, "Hee, hee, hee, hee" then blow out again. Do this until your contraction is over. Remember your labor nurse will be right at your side assisting you. Repeat this type of breathing until you are 10 cm dilated.

When you reach 10 cm dilation, you will be instructed by your nurse or physician on how to hold your breath and push through each contraction. Pushing down in your rectum is the technique you will use. Pushing feels good especially if you don't have an epidural. If you do have an epidural, you should still feel the urge to push. If you do not feel the urge to push, your physician can either have you wait a bit longer until you do feel the urge, or the anesthesiologist can decrease the amount of epidural medication you are receiving so that you have a greater sensation of pressure, not pain.

At this point, you are now in the second stage of labor, the pushing stage. You, your support person and your baby have made fantastic progress and have spent many hours working very hard. You must now dig deep and find your stored energy. It's on you now to push your baby out. It is considered normal for most first-time vaginal deliveries to take up to two hours of pushing. Keep in mind throughout your laboring process that energy must be saved for crossing the finish line. Sometimes your physician, but always your labor nurse, will be at your side the entire time you are pushing. After pushing for an hour or two, your baby will have descended far down into the birth canal. At this point, your doctor, nurse and support person will begin to see the baby's head coming through your vagina. Crowning is a term used for when the baby's head no longer slides back into your vagina. Your baby's head stays visible because your perineum is stretching.

If you have an epidural you will feel pressure. If you do not have an epidural, you will feel intense pressure and a burning sensation. The burning is described by many women as "a ring of fire." OK, so we also have to mention the poop issue. Most women are worried about having a bowel movement while they are pushing. Yep. It happens a lot, and you need to know that it is incredibly ordinary. I view it as a good thing, because it assures me that you are pushing with your rectal muscles, not your stomach, chest or facial muscles. At the point when your baby's head is crowning (about to come out of your vagina), you will not be moving your bowels. Your baby's head and your poop do not come out at the same time.

Episiotomy or a Natural Tear

Immediately before the delivery of your baby's head, your physician will offer you his/her professional opinion on how your perineum looks. Your perineum is the skin between the opening of your vagina and your anus. It may have stretched to the point of tearing and or your physician may think a small cut with scissors is necessary. (This is called an episiotomy.)

This decision is entirely between you and your physician. Whether you tear naturally or have an episiotomy, you will need to be put back together with a few stitches. If you have an epidural, you should not feel the episiotomy, a tear or the putting back together part. If you do NOT have an epidural, there is a combination of reasons why women say they did not feel a tear in their perineum or an episiotomy. One is that your baby's head is pushing hard against a nerve in your vagina, kind of pinching it. Another reason is when the perineum stretches, the ring of fire feeling takes over the other discomforts you might be experiencing. For those of you determined to have your baby without any pain medication, please keep in mind that this final part of delivery lasts a short amount of time...minutes. I have always encouraged my clients to believe, "You can do anything for a few minutes." Yes, you can!

When or if your physician needs to stitch you up, he/she will give you some numbing medication, so you do not feel the sutures. The hardest and the longest part of pushing is getting that darn angelic head OUT. Once the head is out your physician will tell you to push one last time, and the rest of the baby's body will be delivered. Happy, happy birthday!

Cutting of the Umbilical Cord

Anatomically we need to remember that you and your baby are connected by a long jelly-like cord. This is the umbilical cord, and it goes from the baby's belly to your placenta. The umbilical cord contains two arteries and one vein, and it is how your baby received oxygen and nutrients while in your uterus. Your physician will need to clamp the cord in two places and then cut the cord. The cutting of the cord can be done by your support person or your physician. If you have done some extra reading about the umbilical cord, you might know that it will continue to "pulse" for a short while after your baby is born. You can discuss with your physician if, at the moment of delivery, the clamping and cutting of the cord can be delayed.

Holding Your Baby

Immediately after delivery, the physician is the first person to lay eyes on your angel. He/she will do a comprehensive and quick assessment that will most likely lead to placing your baby right into your yearning arms. At this point, you and your support person will have some time to bond. After five to 10 minutes, the nursery nurse will take your baby over to the baby warmer which is in your direct line of vision. Your baby will be dried, weighed, measured, given Apgar scores, dressed in a diaper and a hat, given a shot of vitamin K, provided with an ID band and erythromycin ointment is placed in their eyes. At this point, your baby will then be handed back to you. In most hospitals and birthing centers, all of these tasks are done in your delivery room where you and your support person can watch; it all takes only a matter of minutes.

While all these baby preparations are going on, your physician and labor nurse will gently wash your bottom with warm water, apply an ice pack to decrease the swelling, provide you with something to eat and drink, wrap you up in a toasty warm blanket, and offer you some ibuprofen, acetaminophen or maybe even some Percocet. Yes. It is perfectly fine for you to take any of those three medications for pain and still nurse your baby.

CHAPTER 14:
Newborn Care

Is my baby getting enough to eat?

The short answer is: Your baby IS getting enough to eat if he/she has six to eight wet or poopy diapers in a 24-hour period. This rule applies whether you have chosen to breast-feed or bottle feed.

You can expect to stay in the hospital after you deliver for at least two full nights for a vaginal delivery and three full nights for a cesarean section. During your stay, and once you have decided whether to bottle feed or breast-feed, the staff on the maternity floor will do everything they can to assist you in making feeding time a success. Some of the team that will be there to support you will be the lactation consultant, the labor nurse, the nursery nurse, the postpartum nurse and the clinical assistants. If you have decided to breast-feed, then your nurse will remind you about every two to three hours that it is time to nurse your baby. If you are bottle feeding, then your nurse will tell you that it is time to feed your baby about every three to four hours. Lucky you ... the nurses will even wake you up throughout the night.

Moms who choose to bottle feed need to pack a comfortable, tight-fitting sports bra to wear right after delivery, and then keep it on 24/7 for a few days. Holding your breasts snug in a sports bra will aid in preventing the milk production that will naturally occur. (Even without nursing your baby, you will produce some milk.) Your doctor does not prescribe any medication that prevents or stops your milk production. The goal is to let as little breast milk as possible leak out, so your body knows to stop producing more.

Along with wearing your sports bra 24/7, you will want to diminish stimulation to your breasts as much as possible. For example, do not hold your baby's face close to your breasts, and when you shower, try and back up to the shower instead of facing the shower. Allowing the warm water to bead down onto your chest can cause a "let down" of your breast milk, and again, you are trying to prevent milk from leaking out. Your breasts will feel sore when you are trying to suppress your milk production, and you might need to take some form of pain relief such as ibuprofen or acetaminophen. It can also be very soothing to place a bag of frozen peas or corn on top of your breasts over your bra.

With breast or bottle feeding, before you go home, the hospital pediatrician or the pediatrician you have chosen will give you instructions that will help you in knowing how often you need to feed your baby once you get back home. Most babies will be allowed to feed on demand. The very best way to learn how to feed your baby is by having your baby in your arms. You WILL get a great deal of

THE BIG DAY

support while you're in the hospital with feeding, and you will gain the confidence you need to feel ready by the time you go home.

If you have chosen to breast-feed your baby, your supply of breast milk depends on three basic concepts:

1. The first is "demand and supply." If your baby needs, wants or is demanding to nurse every three hours, then your body will produce enough breast milk for feedings every three hours.

2. Second you must consider your own nutritional intake. While you continue to nurse your baby, you will need to increase your calories by about 500 per day. Make sure you are eating healthy food like protein, carbs, fruit, vegetables and dairy. If you feel hungry, then you need to eat! Your body is working overtime to produce food for another human being.

3. Most women will lose weight during the time they are breastfeeding. The extra 500 to 600 calories a day will not cause you to gain weight. Also, with regard to your nutrition, you will need to increase your intake of water. The average non- lactating female should take in 64 oz of water daily. Your goal will be to take in at least 64 oz and maybe slightly more, since your body requires increased water to produce breast milk.

4. Lastly, remember to rest! For the first six weeks after you deliver, your body is going through incredible changes to get back to a pre-pregnancy state. It is working overtime to keep up with the feeding demands of your newborn, AND you are probably going to be up every three to four hours nursing your baby, which means your sleep is limited. Don't feel guilty for taking daytime naps while your newborn is sleeping.

More on Breast-feeding

The very first time your newborn nurses, you can expect for them to suckle for approximately 15 to 20 minutes on each breast, with a short burp break between breasts. If for your initial feeding you begin nursing your newborn on your right breast, after 15 to 20 minutes you will then burp your baby and switch your baby to your left breast. Easy, right? BUT, it is important to remember that when it's time to feed again, you will start on your left breast and then switch to your right breast.

Alternate which breast you start with at each feeding cycle. The foremilk comes at the beginning of the feeding, and the hindmilk comes at the end of the feeding and has a higher fat content. The second breast will contain the hindmilk. If you have a difficult time remembering your sides, you can attach a small safety pin somewhere on the side you need to start with at the next cycle. It is essential to use your resources while in the hospital. Allowing your baby to nurse is an amazing joy, but it is a learned experience. Yes, your baby knows how to suck, because they have probably been sucking their fingers and toes while inside the womb, but learning to nurse is a completely different type of sucking.

You will get help making sure that your baby opens their mouth very wide before latching on to your breast. A wide-open mouth will ensure that your baby gets as much of your areola into their mouth as possible to ensure a good latch. It is normal after a day or so to have very sore breasts and nipples. After each feeding, if you are sore, you can rub a small amount of your breast milk onto your nipple and areola and let it air dry. In the first week or so, your nipples and areola can crack and even bleed. It is perfectly OK to continue to nurse if this happens.

Something you want to look for, though, is blisters. Inside your baby's mouth, he/she can have "hot spots." These are not literally hot to the touch spots but spots where they have a stronger pull or suck when they are latched on. If this is true for your baby, then nursing can cause a blister, which is not OK. To remedy this, you can change the feeding position you are currently using to another feeding position. For example, if you developed a blister while using the cradle hold, then you might want to reposition your baby to a football hold. The most important factor in relieving, or not getting a blister in the first place, is making certain that your baby's mouth is opened wide when he/she goes to latch on, AND you do not hear smacking or sucking sounds as your baby is nursing. Your breasts and nipples will toughen in a week or two, and before you know it your baby will be nursing and all you feel is connected, blessed, fuzzy and warm! (You might even see bunnies, deer and baby goats prancing around!) Honestly, nursing is one of the many beautiful experiences you will have with your baby. Enjoy and treasure every moment of it.

The first one to four days of breastfeeding, it is important to know you are providing an exceptional kind of milk for your baby. This milk is called colostrum; there is not a lot of it, but it is essential that your baby gets this. Colostrum contains carbohydrates, fats, proteins, vitamins, minerals and YOUR antibodies! By Day Four or so, your breasts will feel much firmer and full; it is at this time that you are now producing breast milk. Make sure when you are shopping for your nursing bras, (before you deliver) that you select a bra size that is at least one cup size bigger than what you are when you are about 30-weeks pregnant. In other words, your breasts will enlarge a considerable amount when you are lactating or breastfeeding.

Bottle Feeding

If you have chosen to bottle feed your baby, here are some helpful hints. Most hospitals have a variety of formula and will provide this to you, along with the bottles and nipples your baby needs while in the hospital.

Choose a formula type. Your formula preference can be dependent on a few things. For example, if you are trying to feed your baby something that is very close to breast milk, then your pediatrician will likely recommend Enfamil or Similac. Research tells us that the content of these two formulas is similar to breastmilk. Enfamil and Similac themselves come in many forms (powder, ready to feed, etc.) and contain slightly different ingredients.

A second factor in choosing formula is the amount of money you can afford to spend. Baby formula is expensive, some more expensive than others. Shop around and price some different formulas, so you get an idea ahead of time (before your baby is born). I do not recommend purchasing an enormous amount of formula before you deliver, because occasionally, your baby might not tolerate the specific type you purchased.

This brings up an important subject: milk or formula intolerance. While you are still in the hospital, your nurses will be closely monitoring how your baby is tolerating their feedings. With an intolerance, the hospital staff looks for excessive vomiting, irritability, gas and basically an unhappy baby. The pediatrician will also be kept informed on how your baby is acting during and after each feeding.

If your baby doesn't show signs of intolerance while he/she is in the hospital and begins to show signs once you get back home, you will need to notify your pediatrician immediately. At that time, you will be given instructions on what to feed your baby. DO NOT change your baby's formula without informing your pediatrician first. Most babies will drink their formula room temperature or slightly warm. NEVER heat the formula in the microwave, and always test it on your wrist before giving it to your baby.

The amount of formula your baby needs will undoubtedly vary, but generally at the first feeding, your baby will probably take about ½ -1 oz. Your nurse will be very helpful in teaching you how to increase the amount, and, within a few days, your baby could be drinking 2 to 4 ounces every three to four hours.

While you are feeding your baby, you want to hold them up slightly, maybe halfway between sitting and lying flat. As a reminder, never prop your baby's bottle up on a pillow or blanket and let them feed, and never put them to bed with a bottle. Have their head in the bend of your arm and, one or two times

THE BIG DAY

during the feeding, you will want to take the bottle out of their mouth and burp them. You will love feeding your baby! He/she will look up at you, and your soft voice and adoring eyes will create an incredible bond that is better than anything you could ever imagine.

CHAPTER 15:
A Newborn's Stool

Right after your baby is born, the hospital nurses and the pediatrician will be on "poop lookout." It's not because we get excited about your baby's bowel movements, but because we need to know that their plumbing is working correctly. The first few bowel movements that your baby will have are called meconium stools. Meconium is thick, black and sticky, looks like tar but has NO odor. OK, support person, here's your easy chance to be on diaper changing duty, change the first few poops before they begin to stink!

In general, the first one to three days your baby will produce meconium stools. After Day Three or so, the meconium will transition to a lighter color brown and will begin to have an odor. Up to this point, any baby that is bottle or breast-fed will have this progression with their stools. Around Day Four, five or six, if you are breastfeeding, the stools will turn to a light yellow. They will be seedy and unformed, so be sure to plug your nose because depending on what you've been eating, Mom, they can be quite stinky! Conversely, if you are bottle feeding, your baby's stools will remain a brown color, and the stool is softly formed. Oh, they are stinky too!

A final word about poop: If you are breast-feeding it can be normal for your baby

THE BIG DAY

to have a bowel movement with every diaper change, and if you are bottle feeding, it can be normal for your baby to have a bowel movement one to two times a day to simply every other day. Many years ago, moms who breast-fed were told not to eat broccoli, onions, chocolate and caffeinated drinks (among other foods), because these foods would cause your baby to have an increased amount of gas in their little bellies, which would make them uncomfortable and unhappy. Now we teach moms to eat what you like, but to pay attention to what you eat. If you've eaten a particularly spicy meal and then you breast-feed your baby, pay attention for a few hours to see if your baby minds that you ate that spicy food. If your baby seems to have a lot of gas or is crying after the feeding, then maybe just stay away from that type of spicy food. Most obstetricians will tell you that it's OK to have one or maybe two caffeinated drinks a day, but please ask your doctor and follow their recommendations.

CHAPTER 16:
Bathing

Bathing is an easy task the first seven to 10 days until the umbilical (stump) cord falls off. Your baby will receive his/her first bath approximately six hours after birth. This bath is a thorough sponge bath. The goal when bathing the baby, when they still have the umbilical stump, is to try to keep the stump dry. The drier the stump is kept, the quicker it will shrivel up and fall off. To promote this drying, always fold your baby's diaper down so that it does not cover the stump.

The nurse who is caring for you and your baby will do the first bath in your room right in front of you and your support person. They will teach you this process. Have your baby in a warm room where there is little to no draft. Place your baby on a towel or two. Do not undress them all the way; maybe leave a T-shirt and a diaper on to start. Have a basin of warm water and a soft washcloth. Begin by wetting the washcloth, and then, with your index finger inside of the washcloth, clean your baby's eyes first. Wipe from the center of their closed eye to the outside of the eye. Change the position of the washcloth on your finger, and clean the other eye in the same manner. Do not use soap on your baby's face.

After you have washed both their eyes, finish washing their face. Once you have

THE BIG DAY

completed the baby's face, you can add some baby soap to the basin of water. Now wash under their neck, making sure to get those baby fat creases. You may want to have an extra basin of warm water with no soap and an extra washcloth. You can use this to rinse under their neck. Use the soapy washcloth to wash their hands. Then rinse.

The rest of the sponge bath is easy. You want to clean from the chest and arms down to the belly and back. Then wash legs and remove the diaper. Wash the genital area and lastly their bottom. Dry the area thoroughly and immediately put a clean diaper on. Sometimes it is wise to place a clean open diaper underneath them as soon as you remove the old one just in case your baby urinates or has a bowel movement. You may change the water as frequently as you need too. To prevent your baby from getting a chill, you might want to dry each section after washing and rinsing. When you have finished washing their body you can put a clean diaper and a T-shirt back on. Now using a swaddling method, wrap them nice and snug with a towel or blanket. Hold them like a football with their head in the palm of your hand and carefully place their head under some warm running water at the sink. Gently wash their hair with baby soap, being very careful while washing the very top and the back of their head.

Your newborn will have two soft spots

on their head. The soft spots are called fontanels. Fontanelles are the space between the bones of an infant's skull that are covered by a tough membrane. On the very top of their head, they have a diamond shape fontanel; wash that area very gently. On the very back area of their skull, they have a triangular shaped fontanel; be gentle washing that area as well. On average, the top fontanel, which is called the anterior fontanel, will close at approximately 18 months to 2 years of age. The back fontanel, or posterior fontanel, will close at approximately eight weeks.

After washing their hair, dry it well, as infants can lose a great deal of heat from their heads. Most newborns' skin will peel for a week or so. This is OK. Your pediatrician will most likely tell you that peeling skin is normal and NOT to put any lotions or powder on your baby until they say it is OK to do so.

Remember, you and your support person will be shown how to give your newborn the sponge bath while you are still in the hospital. After you have been home for seven to 10 days, your baby's umbilical cord stump should fall off. Great!

Now that the cord has fallen off, you can give your baby a tub bath. Most babies love to be in warm water, so that they will enjoy this experience. Bathing is a wonderful time to sing soothing songs and even give a thera-

THE BIG DAY

peutic massage to your little one. When giving a tub bath, you want to go over their body in the same manner you did when you were giving a sponge bath—face first, no soap. Then add soap and continue down their body, finally washing their genitalia and bottom. I think washing their hair at the very end of the bath works best, since babies lose most of their heat through their heads. So, after their bodies are clean, wrap them snug in a warm towel and hold them like a football with their head exposed. Carefully hold them head down toward a running faucet and wash their hair. Dry it well, and then continue to dress them.

CHAPTER 17:
Sleeping and Swaddling

"Babies do not have regular sleep cycles until six months of age. While newborns sleep 16-17 hours a day, they may only sleep one to two hours at a time." (American Association of Pediatrics). Sleeping 16-17 hours per day sounds great, but for only one to two hours at a time sounds dreadful. Hmm, so how can we possibly maximize the amount of time that parents can sleep? Or eat? Or get anything done?

Earlier in the book, I discussed that while you are still in the hospital, your nurse will be responsible for waking you and your baby every two to three hours, if you are breastfeeding, and three to four hours, if you are bottle feeding. At home, you will allow your baby to sleep until they wake on their own, unless otherwise specified by your pediatrician.

There are ways to have some form of organization with this sleep-wake activity. During the daylight hours, "cluster feed" your newborn. This means, feed them more frequently during the day. Try to keep them awake for a while before they feed. If you can successfully keep them awake a bit longer during the day, then maybe (possibly, hopefully), they will sleep for more extended periods during the night.

THE BIG DAY

Swaddling your baby can also help to improve sleep. Most newborns love to be swaddled while they are sleeping; it makes them feel safe and secure, like being back in your womb. Your nurse in the hospital will show you exactly how to swaddle your baby. During the day when your baby wakes, you will want to greet them with a big smile, a hug and a kiss. Then you will change their diaper, and if they are content not to feed immediately, then you should stimulate your baby for a short while by talking or singing to them. Then find a comfortable place to sit while your baby nurses or takes their bottle.

During the night when you feed your baby, the sequence of events is similar to feeding during the day with a few exceptions. When they wake at night, keep the lights low and after changing their diaper get down to feeding. You will want to minimize the time you are awake during the night and teach your newborn that the middle of the night is not play time. (Feeding your newborn is discussed in-depth in Chapter 14.) After feeding is completed, you should swaddle them in a lightweight blanket and lay them down to sleep. ALWAYS LAY THEM DOWN TO SLEEP ON THEIR BACK. The mattress should be firm and free from loose blankets and toys that might suffocate your newborn.

If you are watching TV and you want to place your baby on your chest with their belly down, that is perfectly fine. Keep your baby's head turned to the side and make sure your clothing is not obstructing their airway. As your baby gets older, they will learn to turn their head from side to side and roll over from their back to their belly. This usually happens around three to four months of age. You might lay your three-month-old down to sleep at night on their back, and a few hours later you could find them on their belly. This is perfectly fine. Sometimes the cold feeling of the crib sheet can wake your baby. If you find this is an issue for you, try placing a heating pad on low in between the crib sheets while you are feeding your baby. Turn off and remove the heating pad right before you put your angel back to their crib. Problem solved.

CHAPTER 18:
Circumcision and Pseudomenstruation

Deciding whether or not to have your newborn son circumcised is your right as a parent. Most of the time, circumcision is considered a cosmetic procedure. For example, if Dad is circumcised, then parents may want their son to be the same as Dad. Circumcision most often is done in the hospital by your obstetrician the day before you and your baby go home. Circumcisions are also done for religious reasons. The brit milahh is a Jewish religious male circumcision ceremony performed by a mohel on the eighth day of a newborn's life.

In either circumstance, you will be shown how to care for your son's circumcision. In the hospital, you must sign a consent form for circumcision before the procedure is done. Your son will most likely be numbed with a numbing cream that is placed on the tip of his penis for approximately one hour before the procedure. You may accompany your son while the circumcision is being done if you wish. Most newborns are again numbed with some additional medication immediately before the procedure.

The entire process usually takes about five minutes. A piece of sterile gauze and some Vaseline is then placed on the tip of the penis.

Your nurse will instruct you to change the Vaseline gauze with every diaper change for the first 24 hours. By the next day, you will be surprised at how fast it has healed, and no further Vaseline or gauze should be needed. This discussion is a great one to have with your obstetrician or your religious leader. In most instances, if you have decided to go forward with the circumcision, you will likely be advised to have it done sooner rather than later in your newborn's life.

Let's talk for a minute about our girls. About 25 percent of newborn girls have a small amount of vaginal bleeding on or around Day Three to 10. This bleeding is called a pseudomenses and will present itself as a tiny smear of blood in your daughter's diaper. Do not be concerned; it can be very normal. When your daughter was in utero, she was receiving some of your hormones, although your blood and your baby's blood never actually mix. Shortly after delivery, your daughter will have a withdrawal from your hormones, which could cause her to have a small baby period. This bleeding is a minimal amount and might last from one to three days. If at any time you become concerned about the amount or the number of days it continues, contact your pediatrician.

CHAPTER 19:
Protecting Your Newborn

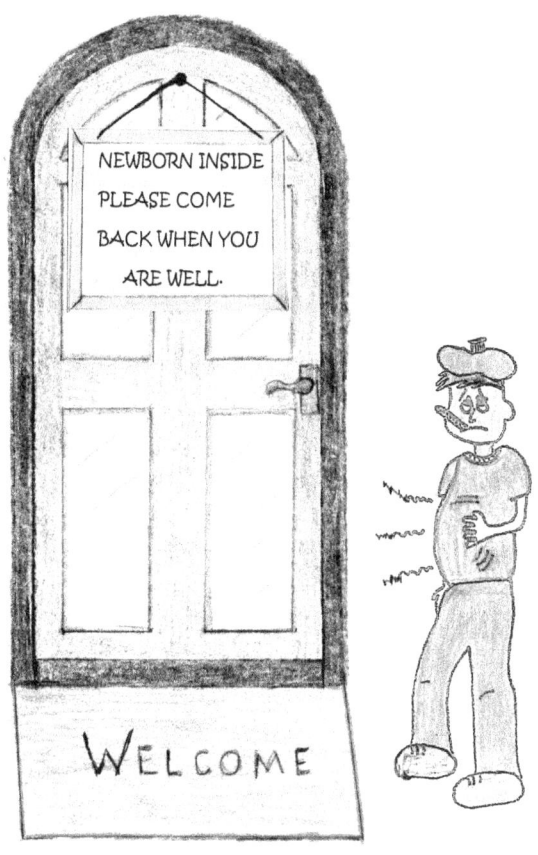

Having a newborn is the most exciting and exhausting experience you might ever go through. You will want to share your bundle of joy with everyone, and everyone will want to come and spend time with you. It is important for you to protect your baby from family and friends who might have a cold or be sick. Your newborn has an immature immune system at the beginning, which makes them more susceptible to the common germ. With time and as you breast-feed, you will pass along the valuable immunities that you have to your newborn. When you do have healthy visitors, it is not mean or rude to ask them to wash their hands with warm soapy water for two minutes before holding your baby. If family or friends are sick, politely ask them to visit when they are well.